Is life worth living?

It all depends on the liver.

William James

Introduction

Most of the conditions an aromatherapist is asked to treat have an underpinning problem with the liver. Eczema, psoriasis, migraine, any stress related condition, PMS, allergies...the list goes on and on. On the surface it is quite easy to tame the symptoms of these illnesses, relaxing the patient, calming the itching, easing the pain, but beneath the surface bubbles a chronic cauldron of disease. The only way to eradicate these illnesses completely is to address the toxicity building up in the liver.

So where does this toxicity we are all hearing so much about come from. The terrifying truth is ....everywhere. From the fertilisers and pesticides we spray onto our food, right through to antibiotics we have used in the past. But science isn't the only culprit; toxicity can also come from emotions we thought we had left behind long ago. Like energetic misfires they linger, holding us back and frankly...making us ill.

So what is the solution? Well, amazingly, essential oils!

Groundbreaking work from the late Michael Cook shows how plants have evolved to do the most wondrous things. This book walks the reader step by step through how the liver has become affected and demonstrates pointers to see what may have triggered it in the past. Written for the professional aromatherapist to work their skills harder than ever before, The Essential Oil Liver Cleanse is written simply enough for even a lay person to understand. It, however, pushes healing boundaries further than most aromatherapists have been trained to go.

It is a terrifying book. Witnessing the assault our livers go through every day will make your blood run cold. But then follows the medicine; the beautiful eloquent and startling plant medicine. It addresses each point in turn, removing the toxins, healing the patient's spirit and nurturing them back on the road to health.

Anyone who has even a cursory interest in health should read this book. Understanding the importance of the liver exposes the roots of most of our 21st century disease. Suddenly chronic illness and thus healing, takes on a whole new twist.

Adapted from the original Jill Bruce Advanced Aromatherapy course notes, the book takes the wisdom of Jill Bruce and Michael Cook and once again builds the rainbow bridge between complementary and traditional medicines.

Table of Contents

Chapter 1 I wouldn't be here without my liver

We need our livers and clearly, I need mine. What I mean when I say I wouldn't be *here* without my liver, is specifically sitting at this desk, here, writing to you now.

I'll begin by telling you a story and as you learn about how the liver works, let's see if you make the same connections as me. Those of you, who have read another of my books *Sales Strategies for Gentle Souls,* will know I spent many years working in recruitment, which was where I learned to sell. The story may seem random, but as we progress through the lesson, you may start to believe that is not completely so. It is also useful for you to know I like baking cakes but I like eating them a whole lot more (*big fat, cuddly momma!*)

My case history:

In 1999, I started my career as a temp controller in Walsall about a mile from Junction 10 of the M6 motorway. A temp controller sends temporary worker to companies to cover sickness or holiday. It is a very reactive, fast-paced job which means you have to juggle lots of things. My day would be broken up into meeting telesales targets to secure jobs for people to go and do, interviewing potential temps and then sending them out to work. By 2003 I ran a contract for sourcing permanent call centre sales staff, and in one drive I recruited 143 staff in one month alone. It's important to say here, *my* division catered for skilled office and sales staff up to managerial level.

In 2008 I was asked to cover someone else's job whilst she went on holiday and went to manage onsite control for an assembly contract. 200 unskilled workers...and the payroll system went down; partly, but not wholly my fault. An admin error meant I had 200 staff vying for my blood.

 The site manager would ring me and shout abuse down the phone at two in the morning screaming about problems getting his staff in. One night he yelled "Get your lazy fat a**e out of bed and come and sort out your mess". Actually, it was his mess not mine so I switched my phone off and went back to sleep.

Not only was I getting it in the neck from the company, my husband was furious I was even taking it since the mess had only landed on my desk because my boss and the controller had decided to dump on me, a job I was ill equipped to do, (unskilled workers) so they could go away on holiday. The two incumbent controllers completely hated me. I was patronising, they said. Stuck in the middle of the entire *****ng mess, I was really very angry about the whole thing.

The week before I took this contract, I had discovered I was five weeks pregnant. I decided not to tell anyone because it was so early on. Since I already had two children about to go to university, this was a shock, and if I am honest my initial response was "Why me, why now?" It seemed to me I had to say goodbye to any plans of freedom I had been waiting so long for, and I didn't like it at all.

The week after the 2am abuse started, I suffered a pulmonary embolism (PE)....a huge clot in my left lung. Signed off on sick leave, I spent the rest of maternity in bed. I never returned to recruitment after being given a huge karmic lesson about what your body does when you refuse to listen to what it is trying to say! I am pleased to say the only stress I suffer from now, is inflicted by me. Now, I can enjoy raising my beautiful son and relish the older kids' university endeavours with pride.

So...let's sort out the jigsaw to find out what happened to me.

Chapter 2 Anatomy and Physiology of the Liver

As ever, I shall begin this chapter by apologising to those who have already covered the anatomy and physiology of the liver fully in their diplomas. Consider this bit, revision. For those who find they have gaps in their learning or were not paying attention at the back...here's a quick recap. There are also elements here, you will find in another of my books *The Professional Stress Solution*. This was inevitable as stress and the liver are so intrinsically linked.

Anatomy

The liver is found on the right hand side of the body located just below your diaphragm. It is the largest of the internal organs and actually, it is also a gland. It measures 25-30cm across and is 15-18cm deep. It weighs around 1.5kg in weight. It is separated into the left and right lobes. The right lobe is further subdivided into the

- **Quadrate lobe**
- **Caudate lobe**

Physiology

I like to imagine the liver as the foreman of the body, and its effects on health are myriad. It has so many fingers in so many pies. Pretty much every system is linked in some way to the liver.

Its functions are:

- Bile production: This helps carry away waste and break down fats in the small intestine as you digest food.
- It produces the proteins which make up blood plasma.
- Production of cholesterol and other special proteins to carry fats through the body.
- Conversion of excess glucose into glycogen to make it easier for the body to store it. (This glycogen can later be converted back to glucose for energy.)
- It receives all amino acids from foods extracted from the small intestine. It then recombines them to synthesize proteins needed for the growth and repair of bodily tissues.
- The liver also regulates blood levels of amino acids. These acids form the protein building blocks.
- Processes haemoglobin for use of its iron content (That is to say the liver stores iron.)
- Conversion of poisonous ammonia to urea (Urea is one of the end products of protein metabolism which is excreted in urine.)
- Cleansing the blood of drugs and other poisonous substances.
- Regulation of blood clotting
- Production of immune factors and removing bacteria from the blood stream thereby improving immunity.

And I thought I could multi-task! The list of liver functions is incredible.

It holds a strategic place in circulation. The liver is the first point of contact for any nutrients newly absorbed into the blood (from the small intestine) and then translates all of their goodness to amino acids, water, nerves etc. "Nerves" is important. Those nerves translate their messages directly to the brain. The liver *should* be holding the body in homeostasis in terms of metabolism, clotting etc...but the messages tell the brain, it's not. Nervous energy > liver> nervous energy> liver, the brain understands "things are going wrong, things are going wrong." In a never ending spiral, down and down we go; getting sicker and sicker and *sicker*.

It's also worth pointing out too, the liver fuels the muscles; the nerves regulate and propagate muscular tension. We have this internal mental dis-ease, but an outer physical one too.

In fact, the stats for liver dysfunction will scare the pants off you! This is a wake-up call to those who thought it was all down to beer.

About 1/3 population in America is confirmed as suffering from NAFLD; that is Non-Alcoholic Fatty Liver Disease. In 2012, Britain saw a rise of 25% of incidences over the last decade. It accounted for 10% the deaths of British people in their 40s. This insidious disease is caused by fat accumulating in the cells of the liver and is one of the predisposing factors of liver disease.

According to the NHS, problems leading to NAFLD are:

- Abuse of prescription drugs
- Diabetes
- Viral Infections of the liver
- Alcoholism
- Overfed and undernourished
- Malnutrition
- Exposure to heavy metals and chemicals

Worryingly though, symptoms may not show until health is seriously compromised. Outward signs then might be:

- Skin blemishes
- Rashes and spots
- Difficulty shedding body fat
- Increased cholesterol
- A thin body and a disproportionately big round tummy
- Depression and /or fatigue
- Cellulite
- Chemical and food sensitivity
- Chronic constipation
- Alcoholism
- Gynectomastic (better known as man boobs)

- Nightmares
- Insomnia
- Digestive dysfunction
- Dark rings or bags under the eyes
- Hypertension
- High Oestrogen
- Premenstrual syndrome
- Hyperthyroid
- Diabetes
- Candida
- Tinnatus
- Hypochlorhydra – inflated levels of gastric juices in the gut
- Gall bladder problems

I think it is worth clarifying <u>fat cells produce oestrogen</u>. This accounts for issues such as PMS, man boobs and oestrogen levels, if you were struggling to make the connection. Liver metabolises fat, (or doesn't, in this case) and oestrogen levels rocket. It will also account for at least some of the reasons a proportion of people struggle with hormonal migraine. The liver struggles, oestrogen goes up, food sensitivities rise.

Food sensitivity is a big area and it does pertain to the liver, because liver toxicity causes it. Whilst I address the issues surrounding sensitivity in this book, the route to dealing with it is covered in *The Aromatherapy Eczema Treatment* where it will have the most use.

Chapter 3 The poisonous subject of toxicity.

Why are our livers' toxic and in fact, how on earth did we get as bad as this? To understand it fully we need to think both about evolution but also the history of Man.

Evolution

Do you like tortoises? I do, a lot. They are fascinating creatures. I don't mean when they are bumbling around eating dandelions in the garden. No, that bores me rigid. I mean how the diversity of their species has evolved.

Darwin based his work The Origin of Species on his findings about nature in the Galapagos Islands. The group consists of 18 main islands, 3 smaller islands, and 107 rocks and islets. Its name was given by Spanish explorers after their word *Galapago*...tortoise.

In the tiny area of the islands there are no fewer than 7 varying species of tortoise, each radically different from the rest. Because a shift in the shelf connecting the islands separated the tortoises many eons ago, each population had to adapt to their new found environment. One population developed incredibly long necks because their food was only growing high up. On another volcanic island their shape changed so their centre of gravity worked more in harmony with the undulations of the ground.

There were around a quarter of a million tortoises on the Galapagos in the 16th century when the islands were first discovered. Then, of course man started hunting them for meat. By the 1970s the number had dropped to around 3,000. What is important to note is: extinction was threatened only at the hands of man. Other than that, the tortoise lives to be well over 100 years old and is one of the heaviest and most evolutionarily successful creatures on our planet.

Evolution of Man

So what about the evolution of man?

Just for a moment, I just want to think about the time line of how *we* have evolved; how we changed to adapt to our environment and the ways the human body has transformed. To save my typing fingers – M.Y.A. = Million years ago.

Monkeys   40 M.Y.A.

Prehistoric apes: 30-20 M.Y.A.

Modern apes: 17-4 M.Y.A.

The most ancient human ancestor Ramapithecus: (pithecus = ape) 14 - 8 M.Y.A.

This creature was a small ape like creature which probably walked upright.

Homo habilis: 2 - 1.5 M.Y.A.

By this time we find evidence of humans having learned how to make tools. Although their face was still primitive, their brain now measured about half the size of a modern day human. Now they are likely to have built basic shelters and even have the basis of some rudimentary speech.

Homo erectus: (1.6 million to 200 000 years ago.)

Here, "Man" was upright. Still, he had no chin and his jaw protruded. His skull was very long and his brow very heavy. Interestingly in the evolution period between *habilis* to *erectus*, his teeth had grown smaller but his brain became much bigger and measured around 10 cm. He could probably speak in some manner quite well now and he had discovered he could control fire.

Although *Homo erectus* first emerged in Africa he spread across Europe and Asia populating the planet.

Homo sapiens: 400 000 to 40 000 years ago

First emerging in Southern Africa, *sapiens* means thinking. In appearance, he looked very similar to how we do now. His forehead was higher because it needed to encase a far larger brain than his predecessors had had. He had now developed a lower jaw and a chin could be seen too.

Socially there is evidence of spiritual awareness by this time as in Shanidar Cave in Northern Iraq, there have been ritual burial sites uncovered from this period. To help the timeline a little more, the earliest Homo Sapiens were what we know as Neanderthal Man.

Finally come **Homo sapiens sapiens** ... 40 000 years ago to present:

(Yes, there are two sapiens, it's not a typing error!)

This means human the wise wise, or thinking thinking (how very arrogant we are!)

By now, we see evidence of sophisticated weapons and extremely effective hunting techniques. Man finally held dominion over his environment. The species spread right from Australia to North America and here we see them creating cave paintings and figures of Venus. To see examples of their work, the earliest homo sapiens sapiens were Cromagnons. There are many archaeological finds of their beads, jewellery and adornments.

The evolution of our livers

That section was long and protracted but I wanted to demonstrate our bodies have changed *gradually*. They have *slowly* altered and morphed to meet the challenges of our environments. This still continues to happen. For example the height of the average human is 3 inches taller than it was just

100 years ago. (Bad news for my husband who is over 6 ft in a town of houses built circa 1582- bumped heads galore!) Average life span in the UK in 1900 was 47 for man and 50 for a woman. Today it is 77 for a man 81 for a woman.

It is easy to consider the modern day human might be the finished article, but surely this cannot be so? We are simply a dot on the evolutionary timeline.

We are here:

The human liver has not yet evolved to meet the needs of all the chemicals it first encountered less than 100 years ago.

It cannot assimilate:

- Heavy Metals
- Petrochemicals
- Radiation
- Electromagnetic energy
- Fertilisers
- Pharmaceuticals
- Some vitamins and minerals

So what happens when the liver encounters these products?

I will add a little disclaimer in here. Those of you who have read others of my books know I do like to back up facts with scientific data. In this lesson, this is almost impossible to do, because it comes from an entirely different viewpoint to the doctor's (allopathic) medicine.

Since almost all clinical trials are funded and carried out by allopathic medicine, we don't really have points of reference to go on. Taking a cynical viewpoint too, those which go contra to the needs of the government and large power organisations are not likely to be in the public domain.

This book is underground medicine really, I suppose. There will be times where I do the coulda, woulda, shoulda lead to this that and the other....but for the most part take it as read. In *The Aromatherapy Eczema Treatment* we address how fatty liver disease is connected to a phenomenon well recognised by allopathic medicine called the Atopic March. This is the way children's bodies develop allergies, eczema and develop them into asthma and the correlation with high incidence of fatty liver disease. In *this* book the evidence is not clearly seen, although it does relate. In the eczema title, liver dysfunction and toxicity evidence positively bursts the spine of the book. Call it a cliff hanger if you like...

What does toxicity do?

- Toxicity sets up dysfunction
  And

- Dysfunction causes toxicity

The more toxic the liver gets, the less effectively it can do its job. Then it becomes even more toxic still.

You should think of organic function in terms of percentage of a whole. If it has 70% toxicity, it will now only function at 30%.

What I should also say here, is we can't blame science for it all. A big part of your liver's problem is you; or more precisely, your emotions. We'll address this in more detail in Chapter 4 Emotions and the organs.

Where do toxins come from?

Think back to your lesson about cells. The cell membrane separates the interior of the cell away from the exterior, protecting it. This cell membrane has a negative charge.

Cells continually die and regenerate, this is the natural order of things. But some toxins have a **positive charge** and so with toxicity, this no longer happens so well.

In a healthy cell, beneficial substances such as hormones, neurotransmitters, amino acids and nutrients diffuse through the selectively semi-permeable cell wall. (Selective: in that only *some* things are allowed through). By a process of osmosis toxins, poisons and metabolic waste *should* leave the cells. If however, the charge of the cell is changed by radiation, heavy metals etc; then it becomes more difficult for the toxins to leave. The toxicity stays and builds up inside of the cell.

Electromagnetic fields

In the UK there is an outpouring of dissent regarding the proposed introduction of smart meters. For my friends abroad, these are meters which gauge and monitor our electricity usage and then transmit this information to a central control centre for allegedly more effective billing. The already scandalous dealings of the power companies with poor billing and uncapped rate hoists is compounded now by the introduction of these wireless gadgets.

Leading the outcry against the meters is Dr Andrew Goldsworthy, retired biology lecturer at Imperial College, London. He draws parallels between how electromagnetism affects water and how it may affect blood.

Electro-magnetics are used in plumbing to combat lime scale in water. Electromagnetic waves emit alternating charges and as such cause calcium leakage in the water cells. Goldsworthy asserts there is considerable reason to surmise the same might happen in blood. If that were true, what would it mean?

Well, if he is right, and the jury *is* still out on this, then the cell actually starts to breakdown and barriers between systems would be compromised. Scariest is the blood brain barrier, but for the purposes of this...the wall between the liver and the gut. One hypothesis is, perhaps too, the parathyroid is affected in some way. This is, after all, the regulator of calcium in the body. Waves *stimulate* activity in every gland in the body, but over time glands become exhausted through long term exposure, and cease to adequately function. Electromagnetics *may* compromise the liver, in particular its relationship with digestion.

Suggestions have been made that toxins and food bi-products may be seeping into the blood and then passing through the blood brain barrier and then entering the brain. This would contribute, not only to statistics like 300% increase of reported cases of Crohn's Disease, but also the unexplained escalation of many autoimmune diseases too.

If you, like many, find this terrifying, visit guyhudson.co.uk to find out ways you can protect yourself, beginning with using a simple switch on your wireless router.

Radiation

Depending on where you live in the world, or what your vocation might be, you will be witness to a larger or lesser problem with radiation. I can remember when Jill and Michael used to go up to Glasgow to shows in 1990's, many people would present with psoriasis type symptoms. On looking at the preparations of oils Mike's dowsing came up with, often there was a trend of oils you would expect to use for radiation. One has to wonder if this might be connected to the Chernobyl disaster which happened in '86.

We are, of course, subjected to low level radiation on a day to day basis, from solar flares, xrays, microwaves and more recently phone masts and mobile phones. Again, this is a dubious area because many conspiracists say the recommended levels are set far too high and, in fact, far lower levels should give rise to health concerns. Hard to know for sure, but when you consider how far off thyroid tests are from the healthy levels, then it probably stands a chance.

Of course, there are one set of people who definitely will need you to remove radiation. Those people who have had radiation treatments for cancer in the past will certainly have debris. Also there are other nuclear medicine tests which might cause alarm.

When I had my pulmonary embolism, I had to have what is called a VQ scan. It was fascinating, but scary too, since there were signs everywhere saying keep out if pregnant, which of course I was!

When a person has a nuclear medicine test, radioactive dye is fed, by IV, into the veins. This is called a radioactive isotope or tracer. The patient is then placed into a scanner which takes a picture of the gamma rays it emits. Doing this, the doctors were able to show me a picture of my lungs; the left lung was peppered with tiny clots which their medicine had thankfully already started to break down.

Radioactive dye has a half life of around six hours which means in theory after that time, it should have broken down and left the body. However, like all pharmaceutical debris, this would remain in the liver.

Pharmaceutical

Michael Cook would always ask any patient he was treating about incidence of jaundice at birth. What would that mean? It means their liver was not working properly at birth. Uh-oh! How long has this been going on?

More, of those suffering conditions connected with toxicity of the liver (eczema, psoriasis, migraine, allergies, hayfever etc etc) he found a large percentage of patients who reported their mothers had received Pethedine during their birth. Tiny little livers trying to assimilate one whackingly potent drug!

You would not be blamed for thinking this residue might only arise from drugs. In a 2004 paper, reports showed a massive 74% of hip replacement patients had tiny fragments of metal in their liver and spleen. The grindings had found their way into the blood stream but could not be filtered out. So, surgery should also flag up warning signs although I can't see how any oils could help metal fragments in particular.

For the area of pharmaceutical debris evidence for humans is low on the ground, agriculture however offers up some interesting findings. In Nigeria there are now guidelines about how long there needs to be between giving a broiler chicken antibiotics and then slaughtering it for consumption. Chromatography also betrays pharmaceuticals picked up from water in the livers of trout.

Remember the question is not: does the liver come into contact with drugs? We know it does, because one of its functions is to cleanse pharmaceuticals out of the body. The question is when does it cease to do this effectively? The answer is as soon as there is any toxicity, its function will fail.

Those of you who have read *The Professional Stress Solution* will also recall we have issues with Vitamin B here. I'll cross this in more detail in the vitamins section but...

The liver is fuelled by vitamin B. Antibiotics drive vitamin B out of the body. Consequently the liver no longer has fuel to run. This is important if you think most of your patients will have had many doses of this throughout their lifetimes.

My GP now refuses to prescribe anti-biotics unless a patient has had a germ for more than a week, presumably since the rise of the superbug. A thought I had about this is: I wonder if part of the genius of the superbug is it can becomes resistant to antibiotics...because they are already in our system. We, as humans, do after all have markers in our white blood cells which remember viruses to build immunity. Who's to say these organisms do not too? Dunno, just one of those weird passing thoughts I have whilst changing the beds!!!

Additives in food

I don't need to labour the point about eating food sprayed with fertilisers and pesticides. I'm sure you get that by now. There is more though isn't there? Think about the depleted soil of overly intensive farming. Think about the pharmaceuticals they pump into meat. Don't forget e-numbers (some of them very useful but many of them not). Consider the overly refined foods which no longer have enough goodness so even their own manufacturers feel they have to add bits in!!! Hence here, we have those people who are over fed but undernourished. Their diet is full of white flour and fats, no fruit and veg and consequently no nutrients are travelling to the liver to synthesize into amino acids.

Airborn particles.

In the case history you may have noticed I used to live by junction 10, land of the air born petrochemical. Now I live on the border of Herefordshire and Shropshire, here they spray fields of oil seed rape and of course our wondrous pears (this is where they grow them for Magners cider!) So therefore we have a different airborn chemical. I am allergic to the stunning rape flowers, so therefore I have double trouble! Never mind, it doesn't detract from my enjoyment of the view of the spectacular yellow patchwork quilt of fields.

Water

We have touched upon this with my poor bilious trout. In fact there are often nitrates, insecticides, pesticides, high levels of aluminium, chlorine and other metals in our water. I write this in June '14 and outside the sun is shining but not more than three months ago much of England was underwater. Levels washed up into farm yards, flooded factories etc....what chemicals got moved into our water systems then?

Alcohol

Long term drinking or binge drinking damages the liver in two different ways:

Oxidative stress

Your liver tries to break down alcohol, the resulting chemical reaction can damage its cells. This damage may lead to inflammation and scarring as the liver tries to repair itself.

Toxins in your gut bacteria

Alcohol can damage your intestine which lets toxins from our gut bacteria get into the liver. These toxins can also lead to inflammation and scarring.

Soft Water

Probably this bit belongs in the vitamins section, but still! In 2012 there were calls for a halt to the price hike planned for alcohol in Scotland. The increase had been planned to stop the terrifying escalations in numbers of Scots who were dying of liver disease. Scientists who had previously laid the blame at the door of drinking realised there may be some issue with the difference in their water. There was. The change came after a study carried out by Foundation for Liver Research, led by Professor Roger Williams, who incidentally was doctor to Irish football genius George Best.

It is now accepted that in areas where it is easy to get lather up your soap, (i.e. areas of soft water) have depletions of magnesium in the water. This is what had caused the liver disease. You might be able to hazard a guess about suggested supplementation! In fact areas with soft water have been found to have incidences of Alcoholic Liver Disease 21% higher than the norm, whereas areas of hard water shows 13% below the norm.

You should definitely be thinking about what the water is like by you and what possible repercussions this may have on your patients. Most waterboards now issue reports on their websites about water hardness.

Workplace Pollution

Some of these again are obvious and clearly you should be watching for them in your case history. The hairdresser who handles peroxides for example. In the same way: what is each of your patients breathing in? These all head for the liver.

In the office what are we subject to? Positive ions from vdus and fluorescent lights and electromagnetism from your wifi are just the start. This static is usually a good place to start looking at the source of a headache for instance....

I think you should have enough to go on there!

Chapter 4 Emotions and the organs

If we move over from aromatherapy for a moment to Chinese Medicine, they are very good at working with emotions and the organs.

Certain emotions find their homes in particular organs. This is covered more in depth in the Mind Body Spirit of Clinical Aromatherapy, but a quick recap is:

- Liver - Anger
- Heart- Irritation
- Lungs - Grief
- Kidneys- Fear
- Spleen – Worry

The positive emotions of a liver in balance are: kindness, benevolence, compassion and generosity.

When the balance tips, then emotions turn sour. Expect to see not only anger but irritability, frustration, resentment, jealousy and rage. In Chinese medicine the liver is the seat of *hun* (our ghost or spirit- extremely oversimplified), importantly here the liver is seen as the seat of fright. Any disturbance of liver energy is going to lead to emotional sensitivity.

You might also want to align anger to the physiological responses the adrenals set off too. You get angry, fight and flight set in and the body goes into an anger flare. So what do we define as anger? You should not only look for the outward signs of anger, often suppressed anger is even more dangerous still.

Let's look at how that might happen.

Trauma

As usual, I am going to use sweeping generalisations here simply to illustrate my point.

Imagine a little boy wanted an ice cream but mum said no. He kicks into his conditioned response of stamping and screaming and has a right good go. Grandmother comes over and says "Big boys don't cry" and so he thinks I am angry but I am big so I shouldn't do this.

The emotion of anger generated in his liver. Because now he doesn't know what to do with it, he holds it in.

There is no avenue for *emotions* to leave through the cell membrane (Remember the cell wall lets neurotransmitters and peptides in, but it doesn't have a process set up to guide out – they are supposed to be emitted through expressing feelings). Physiology hasn't made a plan for that. Actually he is *supposed* to vent; because he didn't, the emotion has nowhere left to go and so its vibration is left in the liver...and it takes up space!

Like a cluttered room it starts to gather dust in every recess,
the odd fertiliser cell from an apple sits there, some

antibiotics join the club...the more rubbish it accrues, fewer nutrients go in and it is capable of less and less work.

Here I will share with you my liver cell too crowded and cobwebbed to swing a cat! Making you sneeze? Interestingly enough that is exactly what this toxicity mostly throws up.....allergies, baby!

Administration

Now because the liver has to do many, many things at one time, if *you* also do too many things it becomes overwhelmed. You know that time around the 23rd of the month when you have to start juggling resources for the bills, signing loads of forms and posting lots of letters. The liver is not a fan! The inability to relax is definitely liver energy; that hip hoppity from one distraction to the next. Which may not be anger, but it definitely is stress.

In Chinese medicine, the liver is the organ of planning and creativity, or instantaneous solutions, sudden insights, trouble shooting. It's energy aligns to that of spring, boisterous, moving forward, powerful. Think of what spring invokes: birth, growth, regeneration, vision, activity, forward movement, upward direction, vitality, optimism and hope. All of these are related to the liver and conversely when the energy shuts down so do the abilities to manifest or feel these things.

And just as Spring does not arrive subtly neither does liver imbalance...it pushes and pushes and will not be stopped.

As the official planning officer of the body, we know liver looks after digestion, menstruation circulation et al. It holds the blueprint to the body and as long as the liver is happy things should chug along very nicely thank you very much.

Emotionally though, what happens if we mislay our plans? We get anxious and fearful. If our plans are scuppered, potentially we go up like a bottle of pop. Spiritually too, it is incredibly hard to move forward in life if we don't have a plan.

It also has alignments with THE administration, authority and being in charge or having to *deal* with someone in charge... or having to adapt to their plans.

The liver governs the free flow of the life force qi. You may recall from learning about the meridians each organ has their peak hours when their energies are highest. For the liver this happens between 1am and 3am.

If you are looking for indicators of liver signs through other avenues than skin irritations etc...listen to their voice. Do they have a bit of a shouting edge to their tone? Are they a bit forceful in getting you to listen to their plan? Shouting is a big give away, because it betrays bubbling anger going on, and usually frustration too. On the other side of the coin, you might have valve-less crying...she/he feels they just can't stop.

Archetype

If you are to understand the emotions and motivations connected with the liver, it helps to look at its astrological alignment with Jupiter. Here I shall say thanks to Jill Bruce for this bit, since it is flagrantly taken from her lesson on the liver.

Jupiter was the Roman king of the Gods. In Greek mythology, he was Zeus. He dispensed justice and authority. He is of course, aligned to success (or wanting to attain it) and ambition. It is about rising higher and wanting to move upwards, not only on a social status but often spiritually too. The lesson of Jupiter in Astrology is expansion. Widening ones horizons, in many ways; spiritually, travelling and also one's girth! Notice the correlation between Jupiter and the way the liver helps to process fat?

Most important is Jupiter's sword of justice. He is fair. He doesn't like things which are not fair. The experience of any *un*fairness will definitely make the liver jar.

Those of you who have read the Professional Stress Solution might also get onto a roll and say "Rising to the occasion-erection" and smugly see the liver, adrenals, pituitary connection. Incidentally in Egyptian mythology, Jupiter is aligned to Osiris who was married to his sister wife, Isis. His brother, Set, was so jealous of their union he murdered Osiris and cut him up into 14 parts and cast them across the globe.

His phallus was eaten by a fish and so Isis was unable to make him complete for his burial. How she overcame it is another magical story. My point here:

Liver depletion happens when you feel as if authority has you by the balls.

One small point with massive connotations:

Jupiter also represents your father.

Key pointers then, Jupiter and by extension your liver is affected by:

1. Justice/injustice
2. Authority / poor relationship with authority
3. Money / unhealthy pursuit of the same
4. Ambition thwarted/ Ambition driven out of control
5. Success and travel/ imposed limitations on these
6. Wisdom
7. Father relationships / relationship problems with The Almighty Father, God
8. Phallus / or feeling like you can no longer rise to *any* occasion

I would be doing myself a disservice if I did not say, if you haven't read The Professional Stress Solution, you might want to order it now and read the section on Yin Disease. Chances are you will sit there agog as the penny starts to drop about why stress is such a social problem in the world today. The striking chain of events that leads from stress...liver...self esteem....and inability to cope changes a person's perception of who they are in the world and what they should be entitled to. That is, what they see as fair or unfair. This self perpetuating circle is giving rise to our society's dependence on the welfare state.

The Domino Effect

Potentially this may be obvious to you, but I think it is worth pointing out here: just as you have the physiological domino effect of adrenals drawing from the liver, affecting the pituitary etc etc, emotionally you will have this too. This is especially true of the liver and its partner organ the gall bladder. The gall bladder governs decision making in particular. You can see how this exhaustion will make a person less and less effective.

Cleansing Emotional Disturbance

When explaining trauma earlier, I somewhat oversimplified. Trauma can be one of the greatest obstacles we face not only to health but our success as human beings. The extraordinary thing about the conscious mind is it *thinks* it protects us against these things. Often it may block out memories to keep our minds safer from dwelling upon them.

The problem we face is the active or conscious mind only actually accounts for 10% of our brains. Inside your bodymind, is a warehouse of things you *think* you have forgotten about. Notice the correlation between the conscious mind and active thinking in contrast to the subconscious mind which runs along on its own. 90% is running amok in the background, completely unsupervised.

Have you ever watched Raiders of the Lost Ark? Right at the end, a forklift rolls slowly around a cavernous space with an unmarked wooden box. Eventually the truck reaches its seemingly random destination. It stacks the case high up amongst millions of other boxes. Some of the cartons look to have been there for eons, dusty and forgotten. In amongst them, anonymous, is one of the most powerful things of all time; Moses' Ark of the Covenant. The government hides it away for protection of the world.

To me this is a fabulous pictoral representation of how the mind works. The conscious mind decides what we should remember and what we should not, and hides things as way as it pleases. The warehouse is positively littered with unmarked boxes hiding all manner of things. Some might be sad, others happy, but many are really very angry. If you are treating the liver at any depth (especially with massage which might release memories from muscles too) you had better be ready your forklift. There will be some heavy emotional lifting to do. Some of these boxes are most certainly going to open.

How does trauma happen?

Well first of all it is important to note they can happen at any age and for many reasons. God forbid you witness a parent's murder, but some children do. Other times it could be short, sharp shock such as having a near miss with a car. Some people suffer abusive relationships which mean they are subjected to trauma after trauma for years. After the event, the mind does one of two things it tries to forget or it attempts to carry on which may of course, sadly lead to a break down.

What's important to remember is my trauma may be different to yours. I might have had an upbringing which makes the things you struggle with mundane, commonplace and not at all shocking. It doesn't mean you will view them as the same. I think the shock is probably the key.

I can't help but think of this is terms of one's relationship with God, which of course again is liver energy. If a person has never held God in high esteem, His loss is really no blow. In fact, think of the paradox, you cannot be angry at God if you do not believe in Him. Think however, of Christ's final wail on the cross "Eli, Eli lema Sabacthani", "My God, My God, why hast thou forsaken me?" To him this must have been the final blow. But in fact, there was one more to come. Realising Jesus was dead, the soldier took one final blow with his spear. Where? I'll leave you to Google those pictures.

In Indonesia, they see the root of love not being in the heart, as we do, but in the liver. In the bibliography a reference to a fascinating cultural assessment of why and how that came to be. I often wonder at how one can become so angry with someone we love. It engenders far more rage than any misdemeanour of a stranger. Love then? Perhaps. Passion may be closer. Anger? Definitely.

In the Professional Stress Solution I cover how strong the physiological effects of a shock are. The adrenals literally poison the tissues of the body with cortisol. The body needs time to purge the muscles of the toxicity and if the mind does not allow the memory, it has no map for the memories to leave the muscle cells. Rather than the actual memory which remains, it is almost like an energetic misfire which didn't complete its game. It's complicated but fascinating.

Please, take to the time to read the paper I have cited by Katie Ruth Linton in the bibliography. It is called Knowing By Heart: Cellular Memory in Heart Transplants. It is an easy read and I know you will find it thrilling. I won't spoil it for you, but...I am going to flagrantly lift two paragraphs, first to show you how good her work is but also to make my next point.

"One such scientist is Candace Pert, Ph. D., who studies biochemistry. Her findings helped support one belief which a growing number of scientists have now adopted: "every cell in our body has its own 'mind'...and if you transfer tissues from one body to another, the cells from the first body will carry memories into the second body" (Sylvia 221). In other words, these scientists believe cellular memory does, in fact, exist...although they would probably prefer not to word their belief as such.

Candace Pert discovered that at least one aspect of our minds has been distributed to other organs throughout the human body. She found that the brain and the body send messages to each other through short chains of amino acids known as neuropeptides and receptors. These amino acid chains were previously known to exist exclusively in the brain. However, Pert and her colleagues have found them in places all throughout the body, especially in major organs such as the heart (Pert 1).

Katie Ruth Linton

Thank you Ms Linton and Dr Pert.

Reader, what do you know about amino acids? Their blood supply is regulated by the liver and so come into contact. In fact in 2012 9 year old Demi Lee Brennan received a liver transplant to save her life. Not only did she get a new liver, she also gained a new blood group. She actually took on the donor markers so it completely changed her blood type, a rare phenomenon called chimerism.

Linton's paper goes on to relate amazing phenomenon of recipient patients having donor memories. (Please, please read it. It's so great!) These are explained by doctors as being down to the immune suppressant drugs they must take for the transplantation, thus weakening the conscious mind and allowing the subconscious to speak through.

Certainly when you use essential oils, this is *exactly* what happens.

What you will often experience in your therapy is a healing crisis where their symptom is likely to play up and it makes them rather ill. This happens a lot with migraine for instance. The weakened state throws up memories and emotions and let's them pour out. Only then, has the original root of the problem being rectified. Then you can start to heal.

What it is important to remember though, is when essential oils work as keys to emotional memories, they bring out both: the memory and the emotion which was boxed away with it at the time. This is good because it promotes healing but, it feels horrible and is very confusing too, because the emotion may have no context many years later.

For example: You saw 10 year old cousin George kick your cat, 15 years ago. After having treatment, you encounter George and have an overwhelming urge to kick him in the nuts but can't actually remember why.

(I say, do it any-way. Kicking cats, he deserves everything he gets!) But you see my point? George might be a perfectly nice bloke now, but you experience the anger of seeing him as a child.

These emotions are transient, and for the most part it is enough to be a listener as they rant. Sometimes though, they are not and of course they may remember something potentially cataclysmic to their health. This is especially true of the liver because of the things it governs, yes anger, but injustice, dads, repression of success.

Time for me to get on my soapbox again, I'm afraid. Yep, sadly people *are* abused, both as children and adults. Please, do not turn into one of those people who think *every* memory points to abuse. It's not helpful to you, it certainly is not helpful to your patient, and potentially planting those thoughts irrevocably shatters families. Most of all it **is not your area of expertise**. Please, please, please if in doubt get them to a counsellor. Keep seeing them for massage and oils therapy to help the emotions and memories dissipate, but do not attempt to analyse or unravel them. This is not our field. Please, if you do not have a counselling qualification, leave their heads alone.

One last proviso though, your patient may have knee jerk reactions to the hurt they are experiencing. It is important they do not carry these though. They may feel they want to leave their husbands, quit their jobs...all manner of things. It's vital they have time to gain perspective before they do. It might be the best thing for them to do to heal, but equally it might not. Do whatever it takes to get them to ride it out, then they can act on the circumstances and evidence later, not purely on the emotion they feel.

Matching the evidence to the case history

In 1999, I started my career as a temp controller in Walsall about a mile from J10 M6. **I had been breathing lovely pollution for 15 years. That was stuck in my liver. I have also said cakes have made me fat!**

A temp controller sends temps to companies to cover sickness or holiday. My day would be broken up into meeting telesales targets to secure jobs for people to go and do, interviewing potential temps and then sending them out to work. By 2003 I ran a contract for sourcing permanent call centre sales staff, and in one drive I recruited 143 staff in one month alone. It's important to say here, my division catered for skilled office and sales staff up to managerial level. **A very competitive job I was always striving for targets and also I had to juggle a lot of things: Ambition and Administration.**

In 2008 I was asked to cover someone else's job whilst she went on holiday and went to manage onsite control for an assembly contract. 200 unskilled workers...and the payroll system went down; partly, but not wholly my fault. An admin error meant I had 200 staff vying for my blood. **Admin again, but also my success had been cut short by something out of my control.**

The site manager would ring me and shout abuse down the phone at two in the morning screaming about problems

48

getting his staff in. One night he yelled "Get your lazy fat a**e out of bed and come and sort out your mess". Actually, it was his mess not mine so I switched my phone off and went back to sleep. **Traumatic behaviour when liver energy is at its peak.**

Not only was I getting it in the neck from the company, my husband was furious I was even taking it since the mess had only landed on my desk because my boss and the controller had decided to dump on me, a job I was ill equipped to do, (unskilled workers) so they could swan off on holiday. The two incumbent controllers completely hated me, refusing to speak because I was patronising, they said. Stuck in the middle of the entire *****ng mess, I was really very angry about the whole thing. **Anger and unfairness**

The week before I took this contract, I had discovered I was five weeks pregnant. I decided not to tell anyone because it was so early on. Since I already had two children about to go to university, this was a shock, and if I am honest my initial response was "Why me, why now?" It seemed to me I had to say goodbye to the little bit more freedom I had been waiting so long for, and I didn't like it at all. **Was grieving and frankly in shock. My long term plans had been scuppered. There were traumas left from previous abuse which had further lodged too. The liver affected the blood plasma and made it clot.**

The week after the 2am abuse started, I suffered a pulmonary embolism....a huge clot in my left lung. **The clot emanated to the place where I expressed my grief, in my lungs.**

Did you draw any of the same conclusions?

The interesting thing though was what happened next. Lying in bed for 9 months made me realise I didn't want to be in the rat race anymore and put me right back in the field of complementary medicine, and of course let my feelings assimilate about having a new son.

Note to the Goddess....whilst I really do appreciate the majesty of your communication, perhaps next time you could simply send a text? Thanks, Liz!

Absorption

If there is trauma in an organ, or toxicity, one of the reasons it dysfunctions is it can no longer absorb its relevant nutrients from food. I shall look at this in more detail in the diet section but for the moment, please remember, it is so.

Chapter 5 Taking the case history

A quick rundown before we move on, so we can check you have all the bits. If you are right, they do have dysfunction of the liver, what is your case history going to do for you? It should illuminate where on earth you start. But what is it going to do to them?

Yep, it will rile them. They will be irritated at your probing; restless you are taking so long, it will almost certainly make them angry. Patients suffering from yin disease (see professional stress solution) already feel like victims. Don't give them an excuse to feel you are picking on them. **You must approach this in the right way or potentially you will get to know your insurance broker a whole lot better than you did before.**

There are two skills you need to drill down here. Firstly explaining what you might be looking for and secondly asking the right questions in the right way. Let's look at the explanation first. This is a vital step in their healing. They are able to see potentially their illness is nobody's fault and understand what might have happened to them. Empower them to understand the process and to become a detective themselves.

Explaining the case history process

Here's what you don't tell them: You don't tell them they are angry! Otherwise you can be sure it will become a self fulfilling prophecy!

Let's look at each aspect in turn. If it were me, I would get the explanation out of the way first then start asking questions. The easiest part for someone to understand is toxicity. So we start here. Explain how toxicity causes dysfunction and everyone is, to some degree, suffering liver toxicity. We (we is a useful word because it implies all aromatherapists, so therefore this "interrogation" becomes the norm) will ask questions to attempt to isolate which ones might be making them feel so ill. The usual places these come from are: (you know the list), so questions about medicines, operations, work, food all pertain to this. Feel free to explain toxins are effectively poisons to their body. Do not use the word poison unless you have explained the toxicity / poison parallel otherwise they may panic about vendettas of arsenic and cyanide. Poison however is a much more powerful and easy word for them to understand.

Then go on to explain how some emotions become trapped in organs and refuse to move on. This is often caused by upsets in the past or sometimes by a trauma they may have experienced which has shocked them, perhaps more than they know.

Describe how the chakras work. Energetic wheels vitalise the organs but are also affected by emotions too. Everyone also has an energetic field around them which could possibly be damaged and so you will be feeling to see if there are tears there.

Explain how illness can come from something as simple as a vertebrae pressing on a nerve which sends pain messages to the organ which then sends them to the brain. Because of this you will want to look at the alignment of their spine.

Lastly relate how each week, as they heal they may find symptoms or emotions get worse. This is because the body and mind are filtering these things out; getting to the root of the treatment. The essential oils will unlock memories, they will move toxins on and of course these have to come out of the body somehow. It might be crying, rashes, diarrhoea, headaches; a whole host of delightful things. Ensure they understand the healing crisis is rare but good. If it happens, even if it makes them feel c**p., It shows their body is preparing to get better, and whilst it might be tempting for them to discontinue treatment, this crisis is a signal it is even more important to carry on.

It will be very useful for them to note down their feelings and findings each day, because these can give you real pointers as to which oils potentially hit the spot. It also helps to write things down because it uses a different part of the brain to that processing the emotion. It helps us to distance our self from the feeling, analyse it and view it from a different perspective.

Gaining information

So, if you have done the preparation work effectively, your patient should understand you are on their side and so trust they can work with you, to get to the facts. How effectively you do the next bit will determine if you are a good healer or a really great one. You need to ask the right questions, in the right way at the right time.

This is covered in a lot more detail in *Sales Strategies for Gentle Souls* because I see it as a fundamental part of successful communications. Here is an overview but for the master class I shall refer you there.

Open questions

There are two types of question. Use the right one and you will get great answers to move your therapy forward, every step you go through the case history

Open questions are designed to glean information. If you can remember back to school you will recall learning to write a newspaper article. All the answers to the open questions should have been in the opening paragraph.

They are:

- Who?
- Why?
- What?
- Where?
- When?
- Which?

You kind of need to turn yourself into an inquisitive 3 year old.

Closed questions

Closed questions by opposition elicit yes and no. They begin with do you, would you, could you etc....I only ever use these to monitor feedback and drill down on a point. So for example, see how the open questions are highlighted in bold italics.

I know what your job is now, but ***what*** other jobs have you done in the past?

"I have been a cleaner, a hairdresser and a beautician"

Ok good, so let's look at each one in turn.

Where did you clean?

In a factory.

Cool ***what*** did they make?

They used to cast brass letter boxes.

What specifically did you clean?

The toilets, the canteen and I used to mop around the furnaces because they were filthy.

What sort of products did you use?

Just...cleaning products, Flash or something like that

How long was that for?

About 3 years

How long ago was it?

Mmmm, 2 years ago now? I suppose.

Now we are going to the closed questions to make sure we haven't missed anything. All we want is yes or no on each one.

Ok brilliant, you have given me loads of information there. Let me just check I have got this right. 5 years ago, you worked at a castings factory.You had to clean the floors of the castings room, and you simply used standard cleaning products here. **Have I got that correct?**

It sounds like chemical rich place to me. **Can you think** of any other chemicals you might have come into contact with there?

What about breathing them in? (open question) **Were there** fumes? (Quickly close it down, all you need is yes or no)

Flow chart

If you use too many closed questions the field of questions will never open up new avenues of thought. Closed questions can only ever clarify a thought you have already had. Open questions move you into new scenarios you may not have thought of.

Compare:

"Have you had your dinner yet?" With

"What are you having for dinner?"

And

"Are you going to Egypt again this year?"

With

"Where are you going on holiday?"

With a person who is happy to chat, the open question will often naturally follow the closed question "No, not this year" might be followed with "Why not?" or "Where are you going then?" But if your patient is shy, uncommunicative or defensive the tone of yes/no might completely cut you off giving you nowhere left to go.

Always use open questions to get data you want, and closed questions to clarify you've understood everything right.

One last point before we move on.

What is the effect on a person when you keep showing them you have listened and understood?

Your patient feels valued. They perceive excellent customer service as well!

To make this process easier, you can refer to the meridian, chakras, vitamins and chiropractic downloads which show these concepts pictorially. I have also had this elevated to a huge canvass if you wanted to have an impressively imposing version on your clinic wall. There are links for these in the email that delivers the downloads.

Some questions then we need to be thinking about as we go.

- Were they jaundiced at birth?
- Have they ever been jaundiced?
- Where do they live?
- Have they always lived there? Don't miss any places where they have lived before which may have contributed to toxicity.
- What is their job?
- What jobs have they done before?
- How do they feel about their boss?
- What does their family look like?

- Do they still see all the members (watch for pointers of antagonism with other siblings parents etc)
- What is their diet like? Do they cook or like prepared meals? (A far less dangerous attack is to approach this through their hobbies!)
- How much are they drinking? (You so won't get the real answer to that, but you need to ask and it will give you a clue at least)

Clearly, I am probably labouring the point here, but the case history is king. An in depth one at the beginning of treatment will show up a great deal of stuff. Try to see it through to the end of the sixth treatment. How have you been feeling? How have you been sleeping? Etc etc You should be watching for differences to see they are getting better, and of course if they are not. If there are no changes after the week when you tackle toxicity, but then your patient finds she is volatile and can't work out why she wants to fight the world on a week when you worked with her chakras, that is extremely powerful information. Most of all though, it really is best practice. I know it is a bind and your patient wants to get her back rubbed....but protect your business at all costs.

Part 2 Healing the liver

Healing the liver with food is a two pronged approach. For simplicity I have grouped all hepatic foods together, because you would just make a meal with these foods. It doesn't matter at what point in the proceedings they are used.

The tools of our trade however, are essential oils.

There are many methods and applications from massage to compresses and poultices and of course creams and lotions.

The most effective method I have found is to double attack with oils rubbed onto meridians in order to stimulate the acupressure points to clean the liver. What I should also add here is one of the effective ways to shove emotional residue out of an organ is using acupuncture so this is a very efficient method.

Compresses and poultices also work very well. Alternating hot and cold compresses with your oils causes a suction pump effect to pull toxicity out. I usually put hot water bottles and frozen peas on top of mine to improve the effects. Leave each one on the back, over the liver, for about 5 minutes. Alternate the hot/cold cycle about half a dozen times. For any of you who have not done compresses before, a warning. Make sure you wash your towels immediately. The salts drawn through very quickly rot the fabric.

Chapter 6 The Essential Oil Liver Cleanse

Hepatic Oils to cleanse and support the liver

Rosemary* – *Rosmarinus officianalis (*Neurotoxic, avoid in cases of epilepsy and psychotic states)*

Eucalyptus – *Eucalyptus globulus*

Carrot seed – *Daucus carota*

Peppermint – *Mentha piperita*

Chamomile maroc – *Chamomile maroc*

Cypress- *Cupressus semperivens*

Lemon – *Citrus limone*

Thyme – *Thymus vulgaris*

To Flush out toxicity

Juniper – *Juniperus communis*

Fennel – *Foeniculum vulgare*

Essential oils to remove Environmental Pollutants
Organic Toxins

Oakmoss Resin - *Evernia Prunastri* (restricted to 0.1%)

Fertilisers

Oakmoss Resin- *Evernia Prunastri*

Peroxides

Oakmoss Resin - *Evernia Prunastri*

Bay - *Laurus nobilis*

Lemon Verbena - *Aloysia triphylla*

Pharmaceutical Debris

Anaesthetic

Benzoin- *Styrax Styacaceae*

Amber Oil– Not actually a plant obviously, so I don't think it has a Latin name although I may be wrong

Neroli - *Citrus aurantium subsp. amara*

Antibiotic

Benzoin *Styrax benzoin*

Amber

Angelica *Angelica archangelica*

Roman Chamomile –*Anthemis nobilis*

Parley Seed- *Petroselinum Sativum*

Anti-Inflammatory

Benzoin *Styrax benzoin*

Angelica – *Angelica archangelica*

Parsley Seed- *Petroselenium sativum*

Sedative

Benzoin -*Styrax benzoin*

Cajuput – *Maleleuca leucadendron*

Ginger- *Zingiber officinalis*

Angelica- *Angelica archangelica*

Digestive Cleanser

Benzoin - *Styrax benzoin*

Basil- *Ocimum basilicum*

Bay-*Laurus nobilis*

Black Pepper – *Piper nigrum*

Cardamom *Elettaria cardamomum*

Cinnamon Leaf - *Cinnamomum zeylanicum*

Clove - *Syzygium aromaticum*

Coriander - *Coriandrum sativum*

Cumin *Cuminum Cyminum*

Oregano *Origanum vulgare*

Parsley Leaf *Petroselinum sativum*

Parsley Seed *Petroselinum sativum*

Essential oils to clear environmental conditions

Essential oils for radiation

Garlic - *Allium sativum*

Onion (to a far lesser extent) *Allium cepa*

Eucalyptus- *Eucalyptus globulus*

Basil - *Ocimum basilicum*

Essential oils to clear Petrochemicals

Amber

Benzoin *Styrax benzoin*

Citronella - *Cymbopogon Nardus*

Cypress – *Cupressus semperivens*

Camphor - *Cinnamomum camphora*

Best to use these in combinations of two.

Essential oils to clear heavy metal poisoning

Cajuput - *Maleleuca leucadendron*

Citronella - *Cymbopogon Nardus*

Aniseed *Pimpinella anisum* – from food

Basil – *Ocimum basilicum*- soil composition

Bay- *Laurus nobilis* – balances ecology

Oils for emotions pertaining to the liver

To lift trauma - Amber

Conflict with God – White Birch- *Betula alba*

Anger - Sage*- Fierce violent wrath.(*Contraindicated in women-causes heavy bleeding) – *Salvia officinalis*

Ylang ylang - regains balance and perspective; helps to "let go"- *Cananga odorata*

Annoyance – *Camomile Maroc*

Contempt – Rosemary *Rosmarinus officianalis* calms the need for revenge

Disgust - Violet Leaf – *Viola odorata* - Opens areas of the mind that have been closed

Irritation – Sandalwood – *Santalum album*

Acupressure

Locations of these are best found by consulting your diagrams on the download at http://www.buildyourownreality.com/meridians

How you use this is up to you. Implement points along the entire meridian into full body massage or simple integrate certain points into daily treatments with creams and lotions. It is also perfectly acceptable to choose one point to stimulate for around 30 seconds each day. Do be cautious of overstimulation. Acupressure is powerful therapy in its own right, and then you are adding essential oils to it too.

The most powerful ones for you to use together are 1-5, which work together to try and get some substance back into your patient's life plan. The liver is the official of planning and when these five points are used together it almost works like "Pick yourself up, brush yourself off and start all over again". Think of it like a very brusque English school ma'am, "Enough of this nonsense you simply have to get on with it girl" and actually that short sharp kick up the backside does your patient wonders. Rather than letting them stew in their anger it helps them gather their internal qi and get some momentum into getting better again; channel it if you like.

Liver and gall bladder always work in tandem so try to match one organ for another; I usually work the gall bladder points on the outside of the leg.

LV 1 - Da Dun
English Name: Large Pile

Location: On the big toe, just on the skin part, next to the corner of the nail.

Benefits: Using this point stimulates assertiveness, discerning when to go along with others and when to assert oneself. It is the point of self-esteem. This is also the point to help a person to start planning his/her way out of their illness; to create a plan. More importantly this point helps them to see worth in their plan.

LV 2 Xing Jian

English Name Moving Between
Location: On the foot, between the big toe and the second toe, a half cun from the margin of the webs of the toes.

Use: Reduce, so move your finger in counter clockwise direction over this point.

This is a nice point to help patients deal more capably with obstacles in their treatment. Think of it as a side step or a contingency plan for them. In their present mood (angry to some degree) even the smallest set back can make them go up like an inferno. This point gives them a degree of humour to smile and see another way forward or perhaps an alternative point of view.

Use this point only when there is heat. You might notice your client red in the face or their skin feels hot to the touch. This is particularly useful if the anger comes to the surface, or if they are feeling warm from prolonged anger (not from exertion). You should avoid use of this point if the patient is weak or low on energy.

Benefits: Heals effects on the body of too much anger.

LV 3 Tai Chong

English Name Great Surge
Location: On the foot, on the line between the big toe and the second toe. The point is located about 3 finger widths from the edge, in the depression the size of a finger tip you can feel there.

Use: Reduce, so move your finger in counter clockwise direction over this point.

This is not a point to use if your patient is feeling weak or has depressed energy.

Benefits: This point pours oils on troubled waters. It relaxes and unblocks emotions (especially repressed anger) and helps to lift related depression.

LV 4 Zhong Feng

English Name Mound Center

Close to the ankle, on the inside of the leg.

I like to imagine this as the point of purpose, or the ability to see one's purpose. At a time when your patient is potentially looking for a reason why things have happened...a karmic purpose if you like. It helps them to alter their attention from blame to "what have I learned?" It also enables them to feel self acknowledgement, rather than having to look outwards for applause. This is a very powerful tool.

LV 5 Li Gou

English Name Woodworm Canal

The name here is a clue to the feeling this restores. Imagine insects crawling over your flesh then removing them, dumping them in a ditch and walking away. This point is relief from irritation and aggravation.

Chapter 7 Diet

This is very much a duplication of part of the medicine in The Professional Stress Solution because stress completely drains the strength of the liver. I think it is worth repeating in both books because it although it duplicates it helps you as a reader to see the cross over. Plus, I am of course that lazy!

Diet

As we are cleaning the body, we need to both move the debris from the gut but also give the body a well earned rest. The majority of the 21st century food is overly refined and also laden with the heavy metals which enabled the retailers to get them to the optimum number of tables: fertilisers, petrochemicals and the like.

Organic is always going to be better (or home grown is best) but it comes at a price tag which some can ill afford. So what I will say is this. Eating fresh fruit and vegetables and whole grains is the most important thing. If going organic is going to be prohibitive...never mind. We have essential oils at our disposal to sort that out. Having said that: if you are shopping for taste, metal free tastes better hands down.

After the liver has been cleansed we need to choose a diet which will fortify it too. In stress terms this is the one we would choose for someone who has been worn down by **Long Term Stress.**

This is quite complex and although I have put them into separate sections I suggest you read it in conjunction with the section on vitamins and minerals.

If you think back to your lessons about digestion you may remember learning about amino acids which are the building blocks for life. Remember these are both synthesized and regulated by the liver. At this point in a patient's illness production is very weak and so leeches strength from pretty much every system in the body. We begin by looking at these.

There are two types of amino acids, these are essential and non-essential. The essential acids isoleucine, leucine, lysine, methionine, phenylalanine, threonine, tryptophan and valine *should* be synthesised through diet. The problem is if there is too much toxification in the liver from heavy metals et al, they can no longer do that.

Since amino acids play a large part in immunity, cell regeneration healthy skin, hair and nails, there are connotations to how your patient may be looking too. They also help your body to produce vital enzymes and hormones, including insulin and glucagon that help regulate blood sugar and stop you storing excess fat, so again we can see an obvious link there too.

So for the most part we are looking at choosing foods which will help them to rebuild these amino acids and also supplementing them to give them a boost too.

The best food type for this is red meat. Really you should aim to have 3 servings a day for three weeks. If that seems too heavy, go for two and some white meat too. Remember it need not be beef, it could be bacon, pork, ham, venison, game etc

Now, unfortunately this diet will be contraindicated in 2 groups. The first is obvious, those who do not eat meat. The second is those people who have liver disease rather than dysfunction so things like hepatitis, cirrhosis etc. Their bodies do not process amino acids in the same way and so leave recommendations about their diet squarely at the doctor's door.

For those who do not eat meat, I suggest three good portions of legumes a day. These are excellent sources of protein and of course do not have the fat.

There are various plants which will help your patient to detoxify and strengthen too. Many of course you may guess because their effects are also found in hepatic essential oils. Most have quite a bitter taste and so are best used as parts of a meal, rather than the whole. Actually too, from an English point of view there are some obvious matches like roast beef, carrots and horseradish, lamb and mint.

Clearly since the aim of the list is to show you the liver enhancing foods, the uses are very repetitive, so apologies for that!

- **Apple** – *Gently diuretic and lowers cholesterol*
- **Artichoke** – *Detoxifies the liver by dieresis. Improves secretion of bile, and also aids the digestion of fat.*
- **Avocado** – *Lowers blood cholesterol and contains amino acids (watch the calories with this one though)*
- **Bitter Salad leaves such as chicory** –*Bitter leaves have an active constituent which stimulates the liver. You can also find this in dandelion, endive, chard and chervil.*
- **Carrots** – *Overall hepatic tonic*
- **Celery** – *General tonic*
- **Chamomile** – *Stimulates liver function and encourages bile flow*
- **Chive** – *Prevent clotting, lowers cholesterol through the body*
- **Elder-** *Regulates bile flow*
- **Grapefruit** – *Stimulates appetite and the liver*
- **Grapes** – *Enhances liver function and bile flow*
- **Horseradish** – *Promotes bile flow*
- **Lemon** – *reduces cholesterol levels and helps to cut through fat*

- **Lentils** – *Makes an excellent part of cholesterol lowering diets because is protein rich*
- **Mint** – *Generally hepatic plant and also cuts through fats*
- **Nettle** – *Regulates bile flow*
- **Oats-** *Lowers levels of cholesterol throughout the body and stimulates the thyroid. Particularly helpful for sufferers of diabetes, insomnia and depression.*
- **Orange** –*Stimulates the liver*
- **Parsley-** *Regulates bile flow*
- **Plums** – *Supports liver function and reduces cholesterol.*
- **Prunes** - *Supports liver function and reduces cholesterol.*
- **Quince-** *Enhances liver function*
- **Raisins** – *Enhances liver function and bile flow*
- **Redcurrant** – *Its anti-inflammatory effects help liver problems*
- **Rosemary** - *Stimulates production and flow of bile.*
- **Rye** – *Reduces viscosity in the blood*
- **Salsify** – *Detoxifies and improves both liver and kidney function*
- **Seaweed** – *Reduces cholesterol and thins the blood*
- **Spring onions** – *Prevents clotting and build ups of cholesterol*

- **Strawberries** – *enhances liver and gall bladder function*
- **Walnuts**- *Reduce cholesterol*

Foods to avoid

Try to get your patient to omit alcohol, fatty food, fatty meats, tobacco, and cut down on dairy.

Vitamin therapy

Ok, so we know vitamins and minerals are vital on a number of fronts. Your patients system is in a state of collapse so we have to nourish it. The very best way of doing this is to implement some vitamin and mineral therapy.

You should have surmised by now vitamin B is top of the list, because its supplies are depleted in the liver. Antibiotics will wipe it out. Stress will eat it up. Prescribe a Vitamin B Complex to cover the whole gamut of healing possibilities it can provide.

There is more. Vitamin B cannot be absorbed without adequate amounts of vitamin C. This should also be prescribed. Be aware of the varying degrees of quality in the brands you use. I have always used Natures Own and Nutri-West which are readily available.

To understand how minerals work, consider them as working in pairs on an axis. If one becomes depleted, the other one rockets up – rather like a seesaw. This is oversimplified as in fact all of them are interdependent on each other. You can see this in the diagram from **www.buildyourownreality.com/vitamins**

In actual fact, the interaction is far more complex as some complement each other and others aggravate, but for the purposes of this, my rendition works.

Magnesium

My beloved magnesium is eventually what made me well after being so ill. When I suffered the PE, I was given a drug called Clexane which stripped all the calcium from my blood. No-one told me to take calcium supplements which I now know they should have done. This affected my already depleted levels of magnesium.

Some symptoms of depleted magnesium are:

Tics, muscle spasms and cramps restless legs, seizures, anxiety, and irregular heart rhythms, migraine headaches, insomnia, depression, and chronic fatigue, amongst others. It can also be a source of problems for incontinence issues too. Many experts suspect magnesium may in fact be the key to Metabolic Syndrome.

The tell tale sign for me was my husband's biggest complaint in life. I am a massive fidget in bed. I have restless legs and as I am falling asleep, I jump very aggressively and suddenly. Then I read this was a classic sign of magnesium deficiency. I couldn't believe it! But yes, after just a few days of supplementing no more restless legs or jumping when I fall asleep. Not only that, no more PMT or migraines either.

What's more, when he was finally born, the child was a dreadful sleeper. I mean waking twenty or thirty times every night. The first night he slept through, he was aged four. A week earlier I started him on a children's supplement of magnesium. His concentration is better and his behaviour is very much improved. It is not likely to be genetically passed from mother to child, but it is definitely congenital. That is to say because my condition became so extreme when he was in utero, he was born the same way.

Magnesium people! It's the future!

And actually it makes sense because magnesium in fruit develops when it reaches maturity. What do we know about fruit retailing now? They pick food too early. Magnesium is naturally found in the largest quantities in leafy green vegetables, nuts, oily fish, fruit then whole grains. Strangely too, when you cook leafy greens, the magnesium efficiency increases too, same for grains and fruits.

How magnesium absorbs and is assimilated is important because people who experience large bouts of diarrhoea will not be able to assimilate it; the body's natural response is to expel it. So for people who are present with problems such as IBS or Crohns for instance you should administer in a different manner. Magnesium is better absorbed through the skin. Prescribe Epsom salts baths or magnesium chloride oil(which isn't actually an oil at all more a serum) for far better results.

The recommended daily allowance is 400mg per day so I prescribe 300 with the hope the rest will come from improved diet. Should we have misjudged and have prescribed too much then the body naturally dispels through diarrhoea

Calcium

You will notice from the chart that calcium and magnesium sit on opposite lines. This is because they are wholly inter dependant on each other. You may remember from your chemistry lessons that elements are either positively or negatively charged. In the case of mg and Ca, they are both divalent cations translated as they both have a double positive charge. What this means is they compete for absorption in the body. The higher the level of calcium, the harder it is for the magnesium to absorb.

On the surface then, it looks like you should not supplement calcium. However between the ages of 30-35 a person loses the ability to store calcium and so after that age, yes it is advisable to do so. Since the calcium/ magnesium balance has a direct bearing on production of D3 aim for a supplement of this too. Deficiency of D3 is thought to be a contributory factor in the development of many strains of cancer.

Zinc

Stress decreases zinc which in turn causes copper levels to rise. Women have more copper naturally and men more zinc, likewise copper is yin and zinc is yang.

Zinc is actually responsible for over a 100 different processes in the body but again edited highlights. It has a calming effect on the brain. If you have an upsurge in copper mood cannot be stabilised. Low zinc is found in patients with depression, most notably those with post natal depression. There is also a hypothesis being tested that zinc may also affect serotonin uptake.

It also affects the thyroid. It plays a contributory part in the production of TRH by the hypothalamus which controls how your thyroid gland works. Ironically the lifespan of TRH is only about 2 minutes as it only goes a matter of inches in the blood stream before it is broken down. Without it though, the thyroid cannot regulate itself.

Now, in some ways we will be damaging zinc *ourselves* in this treatment so again it is important to supplement. Phytates in whole grains, rice corn and legumes all impede absorption of zinc and since this is a large part of the prescriptive diet, this needs to be replaced. (You can't do right for doing wrong, can ya?)

Amino Acids

When a person is severely depleted they may show symptoms which could be mistaken for hypoglycaemia, they go light headed and can feel disoriented and generally weak. To stop this happening, prescribe Core Level Health Reserve and Amino All by Nutri West. Neither of these should be taken during pregnancy or if there is a high likelihood (or wish) of becoming pregnant.

Herbals

Over the years I have found various herbals very helpful in supporting essential oils in cleansing the liver. These are:

Spirulina

Provides key nutrients that aid tissue regeneration and in particular helps to purify and regenerate blood.

Milk Thistle

Protects the liver from toxinas

Stimulates the production of new liver cells

Improves liver function

Chorella

Detoxifies the body of heavy metals (Used extensively by dentists to remove mercury problems from old fillings)

Chiropractic

In The Professional Stress Solution, I give you a brief run down on checking for alignments as well as a diagram of usual misalignment causes of disease. You can download this at **www.buildyourownreality.com/chiropractic.**

You will notice on your diagram of the spine there is one particular vertebrae which might cause you problems and that is T5. Potentially you might have a chicken or egg scenario of what came first the misalignment or the dysfunction but I would almost certainly refer to a chiropractor if I found a misalignment here, in particular. It might be the easiest case you ever closed.

Chakra

The liver is vitalised by the solar plexus chakra

Counselling or CBT

This is a potentially difficult one and you are going to have to use your nouse. Where does your patient's dysfunction come from? Chemical pollutants and toxins, then no, they probably won't need counselling. Your therapy will be cut and dried, clean them, nourish them, send them smiling on their way.

But, anger, well that might be a different story. Also though you are going to have to quietly assess just how murderously they are ranting away. For stress I would suggest CBT, but if a person is really depressed, then that could in fact make them feel worse. In situations of really nasty breakdown, a referral for counselling is best.

Colour therapy

The liver vibrates on the colour green. How you use that is up to you. Perhaps they might want to wear it, use it in meditation or choose green crystals, all help well.

Crystals

Crystals for the liver are:

Amethyst, aquamarine, malachite, bloodstone, carnelian, citrine, emerald, flint, golden ray calcite, imperial topaz, iolite, jasper, peridot, yellow fluorite and white calcite.

Either place over the liver or place over the chakras. Gem Elixirs and Crystal carriers (method follows) also fine tune therapy.

Gem Elixirs

This works on the same principle as Bach Flower Remedies do. Some of you might have used the Rescue Remedy?

By placing a crystal into water, over time the properties and energy transfer to the water.

Fill a jar with water, spring or distilled if you can, but tap water works OK. Place the crystal(s) in it. Put the lid on and pop it into the refrigerator overnight. Next day the elixir is ready use.

In fact these are designed to be drunk, and they just taste like water so that's fine, but they also mix well into your cream bases.

Crystal Carriers

These work in exactly the same way to Elixirs, but using oil. Choose the best carrier and then supercharge it using gems.

Music Therapy

Just a passing mention really to say music therapy is used extensively alongside aromatherapy in the States for patients who have undergone liver transplants. The school of thought suggests the relaxing qualities of the music make it more conducive to liver regeneration

Conclusion

I am almost at a loss as to what to write as a conclusion, because there almost isn't one is there? We can say never have antibiotics again, we could say stay away from supermarket food, we might even say don't breathe the air...but how far would any of us get with that!

The truth is we have to accept this perpetual cycle of cleanse, nourish and cleanse some more. Who knows how long it will be until our livers can cope? Perhaps it never will. What is for sure is we won't know, our children won't know and neither will our children's children. So we have to work with what we've got.

Plant medicine continues to evolve. Our understanding of it does too, albeit a good deal slower. How fortunate we are, nature keep on bestowing us her gifts.

Clearly, now a subtext of liver dysfunction is allergic reaction and whilst I could have covered it here, I feel it makes more sense to address it alongside the illness where allergies have the most impact. It is investigated more fully in *The Aromatherapy Eczema Treatment*.

So then for now I shall say thank you for being with me so far through the book. I feel honoured to have taken up so much of your time. I'd love it if you could place me some feedback on the Amazon page, especially if you could write what you will take away from this book. I find it fascinating which parts touched whom and it really helps me to create subsequent books. I think it is really useful too, for others to read through and think" you know what? I completely missed that bit" and it helps every ones' knowledge base grow.

Hopefully then...we shall meet in another book, and of course please do sign up to Buildyourownreality.com to ensure you get all the freebies available to you!

See you on the other side!

Liz

PS Review and buy! Bye!

About the Author

Elizabeth Ashley qualified as an aromatherapist in 1993, and then passed her Advanced Aromatherapy Diploma in 1994. She has been practicing aromatherapy for almost 21 years.

In 1999, she fell into a whole new career in the aggressive commercial sector of recruitment consultancy. There she discovered her father's second hand car salesman genes had passed along and found she had quite a gift of the gab! More than that, she discovered she could sell...and then some.

In 2008, Elizabeth fell ill during pregnancy with a blood clot in her lungs. The pulmonary embolism prevented her from working and she started to write. Very quickly she gained her first contract as a ghost writer...a recipe book for cheese cakes!

In 2010 she was published professionally for her work on Galbanum oil in the Aromatherapy Thymes, journal of the International Federation of Aromatherapists, and on Tuberose oil by the New Zealand Register of Holistic Therapist.

In 2011 she was seconded on a consultative basis to Walsall Independent Treatment Centre, designed to be a rainbow bridge between traditional and complementary medicines. There she became aware of the rumblings of change in healthcare. Her book *Sales Strategies for Gentle Souls* explains the connotations of this.

Many of her books are aimed at helping qualified aromatherapists to expand their healing repertoire and build their businesses. She also writes for people who have an interest in essential oils and want to learn how to heal. Her in depth essential oil profiles chart the healing properties of plants from the most arcane depths of historic folklore upto the scientific lab trials of today.

In 2014 she ranks in the top 50 contract writers on the freelancer marketplace Elance.com. She is the ghost writer of seven number one Amazon best sellers in the natural healing category. She lives in Shropshire with her husband and youngest son, kept company by their cat, the budgie and many shoals of tropical fish! Her elder son and daughter attend University and make her prouder than anything ever could.

Elizabeth Ashley is possibly of the most published aromatherapy writers you have never heard of! By 2015, all of that will have changed. Elizabeth Ashley is *The Secret Healer*.

Other works by the author

Book 1 - The Complete Guide to

Clinical Aromatherapy & Essential Oils for the Physical Body

Essentially...essential oils for beginners, talented novices and intermediate aromatherapists

Let me ask you, why do you want a book on aromatherapy?

Do you want to learn how to care for your family naturally?

Perhaps you have a franchise selling essential oils and want to know more about what they can do?

Maybe you love the delicious scents and want understand how these beautiful things come to heal.

I wonder if you have started to learn and now want to discover how to build on your knowledge.

Whatever you are looking for this book has something for you.

- Details of how to treat over 60 conditions with essential oils
- Profiles of over 100 natural plant essences and their safety data
- Descriptions of 15 carrier oils and their applications not only for massage but also adding to creams and lotions.

- Comprehensive data of how the chemistry of an oil will affect its actions
- In depth insights into how professional aromatherapists blend...including their 13 favourite recipes from their practices.

Including....

- Sensuous aromatherapy blends by a qualified sex therapist
- Two blends for labour by the midwife running an aromatherapy program on an NHS maternity ward
- A blend for depression by a qualified mental health

PLUS....

10 bonus essential oil monographs and a complementary hypnotherapy relaxation download.

Discount vouchers of treatments courses and products by participating therapists.

AND.... for those of you who would like to contribute, there is a chance to make a donation to cancer research too.

This is my gift to you.

FREE - From 30.11.14

Book 2 Essential Oils for Mind Body Spirit

The Holistic Medicine of Clinical Aromatherapy

Healing the skin, easing the tummy ache or getting someone to sleep is easy with essential oils. Anyone can do it. The joy of healing, though, comes from peeling back the layers of the disease, almost like a detective to find out exactly what caused it in the first place.

Consider this book to be lesson 2 in The Secret Healer Series.

You have mastered which oil to use for what and why...this book takes you step by step though the ancient healing mechanisms of the aura, the chakras and meridians but also explores how that ties in with the latest scientific discoveries into how the emotions affect our health. Using Candace Pert's remarkable "Molecules of Emotion" research, The Secret Healer shows you *where* to look for healing links and *why*.

- Uncover how a certain recurrent negative emotion can be the trigger to make you ill?
- Understand internal processes that mean that psychology, neurology and immunology are quintessentially, and inextricably linked.
- Learn how to use essential oils control your emotions and in turn bring about a far greater standard of wellness.

- Discover mindblowing research that shows the emotions we experience are actually the sensations of neuropeptides triggering our organs to do their jobs
- Reflect on the wonder of Chinese medicine and ancient healing being completely accurate in their healing mechanisms for thousands of years...now that science proves it to be so.

Essential Oils for The Mind Body Spirit couples ancient wisdom with cutting edge science. This is the knowledge the drug companies hope you never find out and our doctors pray we all will.

A short write up, for a book that will change your life. I promise you, when you read the latest findings of psychoimmunolgy, you will never waster another day on being angry again.

Book 3 The Essential Oil Liver Cleanse
The Professional Aromatherapist's Liver Detox

Book 4 The Professional Stress Solution
Essential Oils and Holistic Health Stress Management Techniques for The Professional Aromatherapist

Stress is pandemic in our society.

Scientists agree it plays a quintessential role in how likely it is we will suffer from chronic and possibly fatal illnesses in the future. Risk factors of metabolic syndrome, diabetes, stroke and heart disease are increased through stress.

The daft thing is....aromatherapy can do amazing things to ease it, and potentially aromatherapists could take a massive workload away from the doctor's surgeries.

- Discover the hormonal changes and peptide triggers that change a person's health and mental state.
- Learn how it affects the liver, adrenals and pituitary gland.
- Uncover the strange phenomenon of Yin disease
- Build a better foundation of care, but also a knowledge base that means you can sell your treatments more effectively.
- Improve your healing skills set
- Supercharge your referrals potential from other complementary therapists and orthodox medicine alike.

Includes free bonus material of

- Chiropractic chart of misalignments and potential organic disturbance
- Chart of the meridians and suggested acupressure points to detox the organs more quickly

- Detailed information about how to improve the patients condition with vitamin and minerals therapy
- In depth dietary advice
- Free hypnotherapy relaxation download

Essential Oils are The Off Switch for stress. The *Professional Stress Solution* is the ON SWITCH for your aromatherapy business.

Book 5 The Aromatherapy Eczema Treatment

Healing Eczema, Itchy Skin Rashes and Atopic Dermatitis with Essential Oils and Holistic Medicine

Most people appreciate that the itching and redness of eczema can be used using essential oils, but what if I told you they were capable of so much more?

Imagine if, as a therapist, you were able to pinpoint the emotions that set off these flares? Can you visualise what it would mean to your patient if you were able to isolate the very protagonist causing the eczema breakout and alleviate their pain completely?

Well now you can.

This book teaches you:

- How to isolate the emotions causing the emotional cycle of pain
- The likely food triggers for your patient and the tools to identify the exact times they will detonate a reaction
- The familial traits and links that lead to atopic eczema
- How these links connect with the liver and in turn how to cleanse the liver toxicity
- Vitamins and minerals to cleanse and nourish the system

The book contains very real that will not only transform the way you treat clients, but will skyrocket your clinic's takings.

I recommend reading this book in tandem with *The Professional Stress Solution* and the *Essential Oil Liver Cleanse* to fully understand the cycles and processes of treatment. Add to it *Sales Strategies for Gentle Souls* and your business will stand on an entirely new footing.

Why not save yourself 1/3

And treat yourself to the set?

The full and comprehensive course into how to heal eczema

with aromatherapy and essential oils

I promise you...nothing else comes even close.

Sales Strategies for Gentle Souls

Targeted Sales Training for Professional Aromatherapists

Wonderful things are happening in complementary therapy. Very gifted people are churning out fantastic research and results. The internet is full of what essential oils can do. But when a gentle soul emerges from their relaxing haze of their aromatherapy class room, how do they harness the buzz of energy around them for their craft?

From 1999-2008 I worked in one of the most aggressive commercial environments there is. My role as a recruitment consultant was 80% cold calling in am extremely saturated sales arena. Despite my own gentle soul, I found ways not only to compete, but to excel.

- Learn how to pinpoint the best customers for your practice
- Cost your treatments to ensure every treatment is profitable for both you and your customer
- Discover how to make every conversation into a potential sale lead without becoming a complete and utter pain in the a*s!
- Uncover the reasons why you are not closing sales so you never have to make the same mistakes again
- Create a growth environment where you plan success and always find yourself stepping into it

If you are working with essential oils, and you want to make a good living for it, then you need to learn to sell. What's more, if you are going to say "selling doesn't work on my customers"....then you have simply been taught to do it wrongly.

My dream is to see aromatherapy at the forefront of medicine. I need an army of gifted healers to achieve that. Consider yourself to be my newest recruit and I am going to drill you till you are the slickest, subtlest and most effective marketeer there is. You have the knowledge to make people better, now let me give you the business prowess to heal even more people than you have ever done before.

The Secret Healer has stress in her sights and she's about to make a killing. Listen carefully...she has much to tell you.

www.thesecrethealer.co.uk

www.buildyourownreality.com

Acknowledgements

This book is written in memory of Michael Cook, probably the most exasperating man I have ever known, but nevertheless a genius healer. Thanks too, to Michael's good friend Guy Hudson who helped me put together the data about electromagnetism. Mum, Jill Bruce for her wisdom on the archetypes, and her florid email tips each day.

To Andrew: for his programming and interest in the book. To Aims and Dex: for both just being you and keeping my feet well and truly on the ground. To Anna, darling Anna, where would I have been without your messages every day!

But as ever, gorgeous husband of mine: thanks for tidying up after me, bringing me cups of tea and always being there with a hug. I love you more and more every day.

Bibliography

The Garden of Eden – Jill Bruce

Aromatherapy , An A-Z Patricia Davis

The Art of Aromatherapy- Robert Tisserand

Aromantics- Valerie Worwood

The Practice of Aromatherapy – Dr Jean Valnet

Jill Bruce School of Aromatherapy- Advanced Course

Works Cited

Adrian Reuben, M. F. (2004). The Body has Liver. *Landmarks in Hepatology* , Volume 39, issue 4.

CM., G. (2011 Winter). Active music engagement with emotional-approach coping to improve well-being in liver and kidney transplant recipients. *Pubmed.com* , 48(4):463-85.

Devi, S. M. (2013). *Swadisthan Chakr*. Retrieved July 05, 2014, from Onlinemeditation.org: : http://sahajayoganepal.org/index.php/about-sahajayoga/chakras?showall=&start=2

Did he break your. (n.d.). Retrieved from https://www.academia.edu/2216823/Did_he_break_your_heart_or_your_liver_A_contrastive_study_on_metaphorical_concepts_from_the_source_domain_ORGAN_in_English_and_in_Indonesian#

K. GUGGENHEIM, S. H. (1953). *The effects of antibiotics on the Metabolism of B Vitamins.* Retrieved from The Journal of Nutrition: http://jn.nutrition.org/content/50/2/245.full.pdf

Linton, & Ruth, K. (2003, Sept). *MONTGOMERY COLLEGE STUDENT JOURNAL OF SCIENCE & MATHEMATICS .* Retrieved from Montgomery College, Maryland: http://www.montgomerycollege.edu/Departments/StudentJournal/volume2/kate.pdf

Liver cleanse releases anger from the past. (n.d.). Retrieved from How to raise your vibration: http://howtoraiseyourvibration.blogspot.co.uk/2011/05/liver-cleanse-releases-anger-from-past.html

Mark Howarth, A. R. (2012). *Association of Water Softness and Heavy Alcohol Consumption with Higher Hospital Admission Rates.* Retrieved from Alcohol and Alcoholism Vol. 47, No. 6, pp. 688–696, : http://alcalc.oxfordjournals.org/content/47/6/688.full.pdf

Mataji, S. (n.d.). *Liver Diet.* Retrieved July 5, 2014, from Meditate 4 free: http://www.meditate4free.co.uk/diet.htm

O., D. A. (n.d.). High performance liquidchromatographic method for evaluation of two antibiotic residues in liver and muscle of broilers in Ibidan City, Southern Nigeria. *Journal of Pharmaceutical and Biomedical Sciences* .

Ross, I. (2014, May 23). *Have you got an angry liver.* Retrieved July 05, 2014, from huffington post: http://www.huffingtonpost.com/irene-ross/healthy-liver-healthy-lif_b_498995 2.html

Schoenbart, B., & Shefi, E. (n.d.). *traditional chinese medicine causes of illness.* Retrieved July 5, 2014, from How stuff works: http://health.howstuffworks.com/wellness/natural-medicine/chinese/traditional-chinese-medicine-causes-of-illness6.htm

Stephen I Alexander, N. S. (New England Journal of Medicine 02/2008; 358(4):369-74. · 51.66 Impact Factor). *http://www.researchgate.net/profile/Michael_Stormon/publications.* Retrieved from Chimerism and tolerance in a recipient of a deceased-donor liver transplant.

Universal Health Model. (n.d.). Retrieved July 5, 2014, from http://www.newtreatments.org/Universal_Health_Model.php

Urban RM1, T. M. (2004). Accumulation in liver and spleen of metal particles generated at nonbearing surfaces in hip arthroplasty. *PubMed.com* .

Disclaimer

by SEQ Legal

(1)   Introduction

This disclaimer governs the use of this book. [By using this book, you accept this disclaimer in full. / We will ask you to agree to this disclaimer before you can access the book.]

(2)   Credit

This disclaimer was created using an <u>SEQ Legal</u> template.

(3)   No advice

The book contains information about aromatherapy and the use of essential oils.The information is not advice, and should not be treated as such.

[You must not rely on the information in the book as an alternative to qualified medical advice from a health professional. advice from an appropriately qualified professional. If you have any specific questions about any medical matter you should consult an appropriately qualified professional.]

[If you think you may be suffering from any medical condition you should seek immediate medical attention. You should never delay seeking medical advice, disregard medical advice, or discontinue medical treatment because of information in the book.]

(4)   No representations or warranties

To the maximum extent permitted by applicable law and subject to section 6 below, we exclude all representations, warranties, undertakings and guarantees relating to the book.

Without prejudice to the generality of the foregoing paragraph, we do not represent, warrant, undertake or guarantee:

that the information in the book is correct, accurate, complete or non-misleading;

that the use of the guidance in the book will lead to any particular outcome or result; or

in particular, that by using the guidance in the book you will heal disease or work in any way as a cure for illness.

(5) Limitations and exclusions of liability

The limitations and exclusions of liability set out in this section and elsewhere in this disclaimer: are subject to section 6 below; and govern all liabilities arising under the disclaimer or in relation to the book, including liabilities arising in contract, in tort (including negligence) and for breach of statutory duty.

We will not be liable to you in respect of any losses arising out of any event or events beyond our reasonable control.

We will not be liable to you in respect of any business losses, including without limitation loss of or damage to profits, income, revenue, use, production, anticipated savings, business, contracts, commercial opportunities or goodwill.

We will not be liable to you in respect of any loss or corruption of any data, database or software.

We will not be liable to you in respect of any special, indirect or consequential loss or damage.

(6) Exceptions

Nothing in this disclaimer shall: limit or exclude our liability for death or personal injury resulting from negligence; limit or exclude our liability for fraud or fraudulent misrepresentation; limit any of our liabilities in any way that is not permitted under applicable law; or exclude any of our liabilities that may not be excluded under applicable law.

(7) Severability

If a section of this disclaimer is determined by any court or other competent authority to be unlawful and/or unenforceable, the other sections of this disclaimer continue in effect.

If any unlawful and/or unenforceable section would be lawful or enforceable if part of it were deleted, that part will be deemed to be deleted, and the rest of the section will continue in effect.

(8)   Law and jurisdiction

This disclaimer will be governed by and construed in accordance with English law, and any disputes relating to this disclaimer will be subject to the exclusive jurisdiction of the courts of England and Wales.

(9)   Our details

In this disclaimer, "we" means (and "us" and "our" refer to) [*individual name(s)*] of [*address(es)*].

Made in the USA
San Bernardino, CA
14 October 2016